The Keto Vegetarian Diet

Live a Healthy Lifestyle
Losing Weight

Ricardo Abagnale

0

readers acknowledge that the author is not engaging in the rendering of legal, financial, medical or professional advice. the content within this book has been derived from various sources. please consult a licensed professional before attempting any techniques outlined in this book.

by reading this document, the reader agrees that under no circumstances is the author responsible for any losses, direct or indirect, which are incurred as a result of the use of information contained within this document, including, but not limited to, — errors, omissions, or inaccuracies.

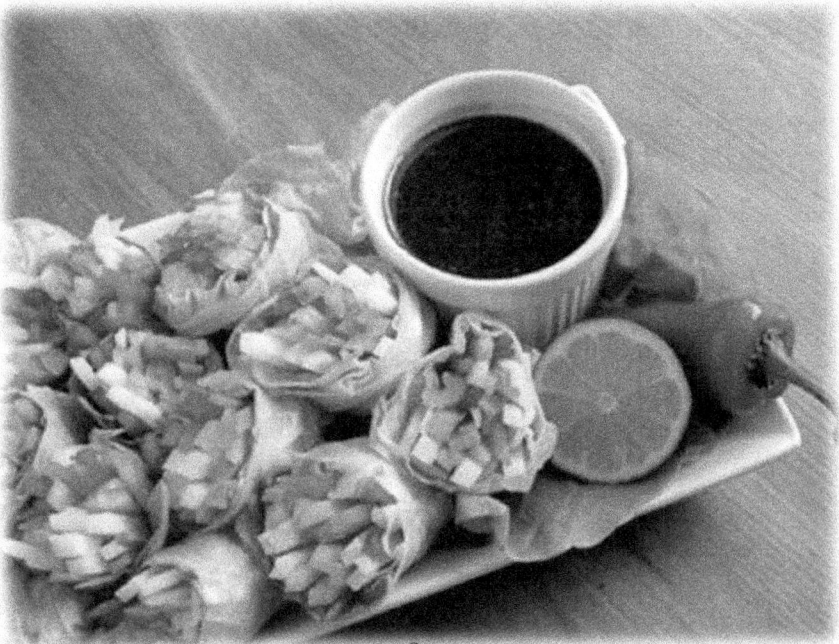

Table of Contents

INTRODUCTION

The Ketogenic diet is truly life changing. The diet improves your overall health and helps you lose the extra weight in a matter of days. The diet will show its multiple benefits even from the beginning and it will become your new lifestyle really soon.

As soon as you embrace the Ketogenic diet, you will start to live a completely new life.

On the other hand, the vegetarian diet is such a healthy dietary option you can choose when trying to live healthy and also lose some weight.

The collection we bring to you today is actually a combination between the Ketogenic and vegetarian diets. You get to discover some amazing Ketogenic vegetarian dishes you can prepare in the comfort of your own home. All the dishes you found here follow both the Ketogenic and the vegetarian rules, they all taste delicious and rich and they are all easy to make.

We can assure you that such a combo is hard to find. So, start a keto diet with a vegetarian "touch" today. It will be both useful and fun!

So, what are you still waiting for? Get started with the Ketogenic diet and learn how to prepare the best and most flavored Ketogenic vegetarian dishes. Enjoy them all!

Scrambled Eggs with Cheddar & Spinach

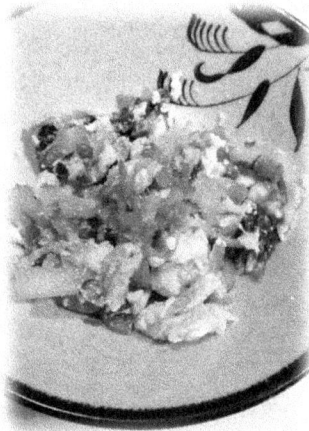

Preparation time: 8 minutes

Cooking time: 10 minutes

Servings: 1

Nutritional Values (Per Serving):

Calories: 700

Fat: 55 g

Carbs: 7 g

Protein: 42 g

Ingredients:

- 1 tablespoon heavy cream
- 1 tablespoon olive oil
- 1 pinch of sea salt and pepper
- 4 large eggs
- ½ cup cheddar cheese, shredded
- 4 cups spinach, chopped

Directions:

1. Crack eggs into mixing bowl, along with heavy cream, salt, and pepper. Mix. Heat a large pan over medium-high heat, adding olive oil. When it is hot, add the spinach and let it sizzle and wilt adding some salt and pepper to it.
2. When the spinach is fully cooked, reduce heat to medium-low and add in the egg mixture. Stir the eggs slowly and cook.
3. When the eggs have set, add in the cheese on top and allow it to melt.

Waffle/Cinnamon Roll

Preparation time: 5 minutes

Cooking time: 6 minutes

Servings: 1

Nutritional Values (Per Serving):

- Calories: 545
- Fat: 52 g
- Carbs: 6 g
- Protein: 25 g

Ingredients:

Waffle:

- ½ teaspoon vanilla extract
- ½ teaspoon cinnamon
- ¼ teaspoon baking soda 2 large eggs
- 1 tablespoon erythritol
- 6 tablespoons almond flour

Frosting:

- 2 teaspoons batter from waffles
- 2 tablespoons cream cheese
- 1 tablespoon heavy cream

- ¼ teaspoon of cinnamon
- 1 tablespoon erythritol
- ¼ teaspoon vanilla extract

Directions:

1. Add all the dry waffle ingredients in a mixing bowl.
2. In another mixing bowl, mix your wet ingredients. Ensure that they are combined well. Add your wet ingredients to the dry ingredients and blend well.
3. Heat your waffle iron. When waffle iron is hot, add your batter. Remember to reserve 2 teaspoons of your waffle batter for the frosting.
4. While the waffle is cooking, add your cream cheese and erythritol to a small bowl. Now add heavy cream, cinnamon, and batter. Mix until smooth.
5. Once the waffle is finished cooking, remove it from iron, place on serving the dish and spread frosting on top. Enjoy!

Creamy Zucchini Noodles

Preparation time: 10 minutes

Cooking time: 5 minutes

Servings: 4

Nutritional Values (Per Serving):

- Calories: 307
- Fat: 21.9 g
- Carbohydrates: 9.2 g
- Sugar: 3.6 g
- Protein:20.6 g
- Cholesterol: 33 mg

Ingredients:

- 3 medium zucchinis, use spiralizer to make noodles
- 1 tablespoon arrowroot powder
- ¼ teaspoon ground nutmeg
- Black pepper to taste
- teaspoon butter
- garlic cloves, minced
- ½ cup almond milk, unsweetened
- ¾ cup parmesan cheese, grated

Directions:

1. In a pan over medium-high heat melt butter. Add in the garlic and cook for about 1 minute or until garlic softens. Decrease the heat to medium-low.
2. Add heavy cream, almond milk, nutmeg and stir well, bringing to a simmer.
3. In a mixing bowl, whisk 2 tablespoons of water and arrowroot powder until smooth. Pour mixture into the pan and stir well. Add black pepper and grated cheese and stir until cheese melts. Pour sauce into a bowl, cover and set aside.
4. Heat pan over medium-high heat. Once the pan is hot adding in zucchini noodles and stir until they soften, for about 5 minutes.
5. Now stir in the prepared sauce and serve.

MAINS

Greens and Olives Pan

Preparation time: 10 minutes

Cooking time: 15 minutes

Servings: 4

Nutritional Values (Per Serving):

- Calories 136
- Fat 13.1
- Fiber 1.9
- Carbs 4.4
- Protein 2.8

Ingredients:

- 4 spring onions, chopped
- 2 tablespoons olive oil
- ½ cup green olives, pitted and halved

- ¼ cup pine nuts, toasted
- 1 tablespoon balsamic vinegar
- 2 cups baby spinach
- 1 cup baby arugula
- 1 cup asparagus, trimmed, blanched and halved
- Salt and black pepper to the taste

Directions:

1. Heat up a pan with the oil over medium high heat, add the spring onions and the asparagus and sauté for 5 minutes.
2. Add the olives, spinach and the other ingredients, toss, cook over medium heat for 10 minutes, divide between plates and serve for lunch.

Mushrooms and Chard Soup

Preparation time: 10 minutes

Cooking time: 30 minutes

Servings: 4

Nutritional Values (Per Serving):

- Calories 140
- Fat 4
- Fiber 2
- Carbs 4
- Protein 8

Ingredients:

- 3 cups Swiss chard, chopped
- 6 cups vegetable stock
- 1 cup mushrooms, sliced
- 2 garlic cloves, minced
- 1 tablespoon olive oil

- 2 scallions, chopped
- 2 tablespoons balsamic vinegar
- ¼ cup basil, chopped
- Salt and black pepper to the taste
- 1 tablespoon cilantro, chopped

Directions:

1. Heat up a pot with the oil over medium high heat, add the scallions and the garlic and sauté for 5 minutes.
2. Add the mushrooms and sauté for another 5 minutes.
3. Add the rest of the ingredients, toss, bring to a simmer and cook over medium heat for 20 minutes more.
4. Ladle the soup into bowls and serve.

Tomato, Green Beans and Chard Soup

Preparation time: 10 minutes

Cooking time: 35 minutes

Servings: 4

Nutritional Values (Per Serving):

- Calories 150
- Fat 8
- Fiber 2
- Carbs 4
- Protein 9

Ingredients:

- 2 scallions, chopped
- 1 cup Swiss chard, chopped
- 1 tablespoon olive oil

- 1 red bell pepper, chopped
- Salt and black pepper to the taste
- 1 cup tomatoes, cubed
- 1 cup green beans, chopped
- 6 cups vegetable stock
- 2 tablespoons tomato passata
- 2 garlic cloves, minced
- 2 teaspoons thyme, chopped
- ½ teaspoon red pepper flakes

Directions:

1. Heat up a pot with the oil over medium heat, add the scallions, garlic and the pepper flakes and sauté for 5 minutes.
2. Add the chard and the other ingredients, toss, bring to a simmer and cook over medium heat for 30 minutes more.
3. Ladle the soup into bowls and serve for lunch.

Hot Roasted Peppers Cream

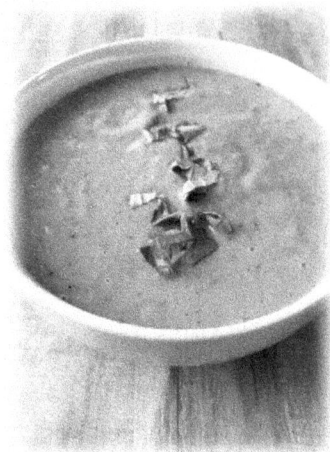

Preparation time: 10 minutes

Cooking time: 30 minutes

Servings: 4

Nutritional Values (Per Serving):

- Calories 140
- Fat 2
- Fiber 2
- Carbs 5
- Protein 8

Ingredients:

- 1 red chili pepper, minced
- 4 garlic cloves, minced
- 2 pounds mixed bell peppers, roasted, peeled and chopped
- 4 scallions, chopped
- 1 cup coconut cream
- Salt and black pepper to the taste
- 2 tablespoons olive oil
- ½ tablespoon basil, chopped
- 4 cups vegetable stock
- ¼ cup chives, chopped

Directions:

1. Heat up a pot with the oil over medium heat, add the garlic and the chili pepper and sauté for 5 minutes.
2. Add the peppers and the other ingredients, toss, bring to a simmer and cook over medium heat for 25 minutes.
3. Blend the soup using an immersion blender, divide into bowls and serve.

Eggplant and Peppers Soup

Preparation time: 10 minutes

Cooking time: 40 minutes

Servings: 4

Nutritional Values (Per Serving):

- Calories 180
- Fat 2
- Fiber 3
- Carbs 5
- Protein 10

Ingredients:

- 2 red bell peppers, chopped
- 3 scallions, chopped
- 3 garlic cloves, minced
- 2 tablespoon olive oil
- Salt and black pepper to the taste

- 5 cups vegetable stock
- 1 bay leaf
- ½ cup coconut cream
- 1 pound eggplants, roughly cubed
- 2 tablespoons basil, chopped

Directions:

1. Heat up a pot with the oil over medium heat, add the scallions and the garlic and sauté for 5 minutes.
2. Add the peppers and the eggplants and sauté for 5 minutes more.
3. Add the remaining ingredients, toss, bring to a simmer, cook for 30 minutes, ladle into bowls and serve for lunch.

Eggplant and Olives Stew

Preparation time: 10 minutes

Cooking time: 30 minutes

Servings: 4

Nutritional Values (Per Serving):

- Calories 93
- Fat 1.8
- Fiber 10.6
- Carbs 18.6
- Protein 3.4

Ingredients:

- 2 scallions, chopped
- 2 tablespoons avocado oil
- 2 garlic cloves, chopped
- 1 bunch parsley, chopped
- Salt and black pepper to the taste

- 1 teaspoon basil, dried
- 1 teaspoon cumin, dried
- 2 eggplants, roughly cubed
- 1 cup green olives, pitted and sliced
- 3 tablespoons balsamic vinegar
- ½ cup tomato passata

Directions:

1. Heat up a pot with the oil over medium heat, add the scallions, garlic, basil and cumin and sauté for 5 minutes.
2. Add the eggplants and the other ingredients, toss, cook over medium heat for 25 minutes more, divide into bowls and serve.

Cauliflower and Artichokes Soup

Preparation time: 10 minutes

Cooking time: 25 minutes

Servings: 4

Nutritional Values (Per Serving):

- Calories 207
- Fat 17.2
- Fiber 6.2
- Carbs 14.1
- Protein 4.7

Ingredients:

- 1 pound cauliflower florets
- 1 cup canned artichoke hearts, drained and chopped
- 2 scallions, chopped

- 2 tablespoons olive oil
- 2 garlic cloves, minced
- 6 cups vegetable stock
- Salt and black pepper to the taste
- 2/3 cup coconut cream
- 2 tablespoons cilantro, chopped

Directions:

1. Heat up a pot with the oil over medium heat, add the scallions and the garlic and sauté for 5 minutes.
2. Add the cauliflower and the other ingredients, toss, bring to a simmer and cook over medium heat for 20 minutes more.
3. Blend the soup using an immersion blender, divide it into bowls and serve.

Hot Cabbage Soup

Preparation time: 10 minutes

Cooking time: 30 minutes

Servings: 4

Nutritional Values (Per Serving):

- Calories 117
- Fat 7.5
- Fiber 5.2
- Carbs 12.7
- Protein 2.8

Ingredients:

- 3 spring onions, chopped
- 1 green cabbage head, shredded
- 2 tablespoons olive oil
- 1 tablespoon ginger, grated
- 1 teaspoon cumin, ground

- 6 cups vegetable stock
- Salt and black pepper to the taste
- 1 teaspoon hot paprika
- 1 teaspoon chili powder
- 1 tablespoon cilantro, chopped

Directions:

1. Heat up a pot with the oil over medium heat, add the spring onions, ginger and the cumin and sauté for 5 minutes.
2. Add the cabbage and the other ingredients, stir, bring to a simmer and cook over medium heat for 25 minutes more.
3. Ladle the soup into bowls and serve for lunch.

Oregano Zucchinis and Broccoli

Preparation time: 10 minutes

Cooking time: 20 minutes

Servings: 4

Nutritional Values (Per Serving):

- Calories 140
- Fat 2
- Fiber 1
- Carbs 1
- Protein 6

Ingredients:

- 1 pound zucchinis, sliced
- 1 cup broccoli florets
- Salt and black pepper to the taste

- 2 tablespoons avocado oil
- 2 tablespoons chili powder
- ½ teaspoon oregano, dried
- 1 and ½ tablespoons coriander, chopped

Directions:

1. Heat up a pan with the oil over medium heat, add the zucchinis, broccoli and the other ingredients, toss, cook over medium heat for 20 minutes, divide between plates and serve as a side dish.

Spinach Mash

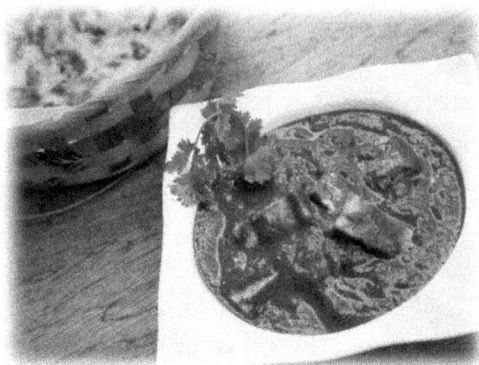

Preparation time: 10 minutes

Cooking time: 15 minutes

Servings: 4

Nutritional Values (Per Serving):

- Calories 190
- Fat 16
- Fiber 7
- Carbs 3
- Protein 5

Ingredients:

- 1 pound spinach leaves
- 3 scallions, chopped
- 2 garlic cloves, minced
- ¼ cup coconut cream
- 2 tablespoons olive oil
- Salt and black pepper to the taste
- ½ tablespoon chives, chopped

Directions:

2. Heat up a pan with the oil over medium heat, add the scallions and the garlic and sauté for 2 minutes.
3. Add the spinach and the other ingredients except the chives, toss, cook over medium heat for 13 minutes, blend using an immersion blender, divide between plates, sprinkle the chives on top and serve.

Jalapeno Zucchinis Mix

Preparation time: 10 minutes

Cooking time: 30 minutes

Servings: 4

Nutritional Values (Per Serving):

- Calories 120
- Fat 4.2
- Fiber 2.3
- Carbs 3
- Protein 6

Ingredients:

- 1 pound zucchinis, sliced
- ¼ cup green onions, chopped
- ½ cup cashew cheese, shredded
- 1 cup coconut cream
- 2 jalapenos, chopped

- Salt and black pepper to the taste
- 2 tablespoons chives, chopped

Directions:

1. In a baking dish, combine the zucchinis with the onions and the other ingredients, toss, bake at 390 degrees F for 30 minutes, divide between plates and serve.

Coconut and Tomatoes Mix

Preparation time: 5 minutes

Cooking time: 12 minutes

Servings: 4

Nutritional Values (Per Serving):

- Calories 152
- Fat 13.8
- Fiber 3.4
- Carbs 7.7
- Protein 1.8

Ingredients:

- 1 pound tomatoes, cut into wedges
- 1 cup coconut, unsweetened and shredded
- 2 tablespoons coconut oil, melted
- 1 tablespoon chives, chopped
- 1 teaspoon coriander, ground

- 1 teaspoon fennel seeds
- Salt and black pepper to the taste

Directions:

- Heat up a pan with the oil over medium heat, add the coriander and fennel seeds and cook for 2 minutes.
- Add the tomatoes and the other ingredients, toss, cook over medium heat for 10 minutes, divide between plates and serve.

Mushroom Rice

Preparation time: 10 minutes

Cooking time: 20 minutes

Servings: 4

Nutritional Values (Per Serving):

- Calories 124
- Fat 2.4
- Fiber 1.5
- Carbs 2
- Protein 1.2

Ingredients:

- 2 tablespoons olive oil
- 1 cup mushrooms, sliced
- 2 cups cauliflower rice
- 2 tablespoons lime juice
- 2 tablespoons almonds, sliced

- 1 cup veggie stock
- Salt and black pepper to the taste
- ½ teaspoon garlic powder
- 1 tablespoon parsley, chopped

Directions:

2. Heat up a pan with the oil over medium heat, add the mushrooms and the almonds and sauté for 5 minutes.
3. Add the cauliflower rice and the other ingredients, toss, cook over medium heat for 15 minutes more, divide between plates and serve.

Cucumber and Cauliflower Mix

Preparation time: 10 minutes

Cooking time: 12 minutes

Servings: 4

Nutritional Values (Per Serving):

- Calories 53
- Fat 1.2
- Fiber 3.9
- Carbs 9.9
- Protein 3

Ingredients:

- 1 cucumber, cubed
- 1 pound cauliflower florets
- 1 spring onion, chopped
- 2 tablespoons avocado oil
- 1 tablespoon balsamic vinegar

- ¼ teaspoon red pepper flakes
- Salt and black pepper to the taste
- 1 tablespoon thyme, chopped

Directions:

1. Heat up a pan with the oil over medium heat, add the spring onions and the pepper flakes and sauté for 2 minutes.
2. Add the cucumber and the other ingredients, toss, cook over medium heat for 10 minutes more, divide between plates and serve.

Sicilian Stuffed Tomatoes

Preparation time: 10 minutes

Cooking time: 30 minutes

Servings: 4

Ingredients:

- 2 cups water
- 1 cup couscous Salt
- 3 green onions, minced
- 1/3 cup golden raisins
- 1 teaspoon finely grated orange zest
- 4 large ripe tomatoes
- 1/3 cup toasted pine nuts
- 1/4 cup minced fresh parsley
- Freshly ground black pepper
- 2 teaspoons olive oil

Directions:

1. Preheat the oven to 375°F. Lightly oil a 9 x 13-inch baking pan and set aside. In a large saucepan, bring the water to a boil over high heat. Stir in the couscous and salt to taste and remove from the heat. Stir in the green onions, raisins, and orange zest. Cover and set aside for 5 minutes.

2. Cut a ½-inch-thick slice off the top of each of the tomatoes. Scoop out the pulp, keeping the tomato shells intact. Chop the pulp and place it in a large bowl. Add the couscous mixture along with the pine nuts, parsley, and salt and pepper to taste. Mix well.

3. Fill the tomatoes with the mixture and place them in the prepared pan. Drizzle the tomatoes with the oil, cover with foil, and bake until hot, about 20 minutes. Serve immediately.

Basic Baked Potatoes

Preparation time: 5 minutes

Cooking time: 60 minutes

Servings: 5

Nutritional Values (Per Serving):

- Calories: 171
- Fat: 3g
- Protein: 4g
- Carbohydrates: 34g
- Fiber: 5g
- Sugar: 3g
- Sodium: 129mg

Ingredients:

- 5 medium Russet potatoes or a variety of potatoes, washed and patted dry

- 1 to 2 tablespoons extra-virgin olive oil or aquafaba (see tip)
- ¼ teaspoon salt
- ¼ teaspoon freshly ground black pepper

Directions:

1. Preheat the oven to 400°F. Pierce each potato several times with a fork or a knife. Brush the olive oil over the potatoes, then rub each with a pinch of the salt and a pinch of the pepper.
2. Place the potatoes on a baking sheet and bake for 50 to 60 minutes, until tender. Place the potatoes on a baking rack and cool completely. Transfer to an airtight container or 5 single-serving containers. Let cool before sealing the lids.

Orange-Dressed Asparagus

Preparation time: 5 minutes

Cooking time: 10 minutes

Servings: 4

Ingredients:

- 1 medium shallot, minced
- 2 teaspoons orange zest ⅓ cup fresh orange juice
- 1 tablespoon fresh lemon juice Pinch sugar
- 2 tablespoons olive oil
- Salt and freshly ground black pepper
- 1 pound asparagus, tough ends trimmed

Directions:

1. In a small bowl, combine the shallot, orange zest, orange juice, lemon juice, sugar, and oil. Add salt and pepper to taste and mix well. Set aside to allow flavors to blend, for 5 to 10 minutes.

2. Steam the asparagus until just tender, 4 to 5 minutes. If serving hot, arrange on a serving platter and drizzle the dressing over the asparagus. Serve at once.

3. If serving chilled, run the asparagus under cold water to stop the cooking process and retain the color. Drain on paper towels, then cover and refrigerate until chilled, about 1 hour. To serve, arrange the asparagus on a serving platter and drizzle with the dressing.

Broccoli with Almonds

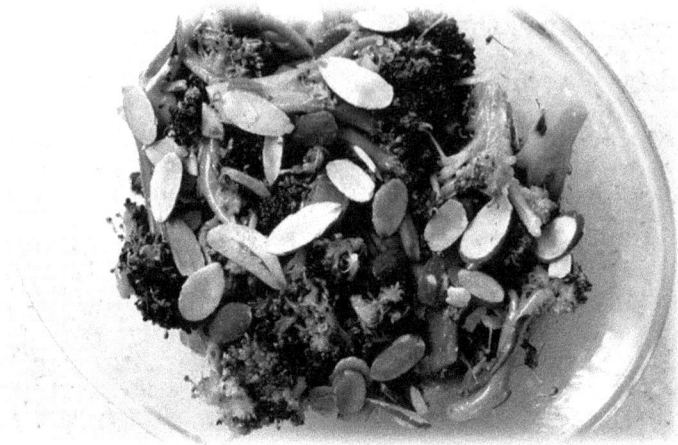

Preparation time: 5 minutes

Cooking time: 15 minutes

Servings: 4

Ingredients:

- 1 pound broccoli, cut into small florets
- 2 tablespoons olive oil
- 3 garlic cloves, minced
- 1 cup thinly sliced white mushrooms
- 1/4 cup dry white wine

- 2 tablespoons minced fresh parsley
- Salt and freshly ground black pepper
- ½ cup slivered toasted almonds

Directions:

1. Steam the broccoli until just tender, about 5 minutes. Run under cold water and set aside.
2. In a large skillet, heat 1 tablespoon of the oil over medium heat. Add the garlic and mushrooms and cook until soft, about 5 minutes. Add the wine and cook 1 minute longer. Add the steamed broccoli and parsley and season with salt and pepper to taste. Cook until the liquid is evaporated and the broccoli is hot, about 3 minutes.
3. Transfer to a serving bowl, drizzle with the remaining 1 tablespoon oil and the almonds, and toss to coat. Serve immediately.

Glazed Curried Carrots

Preparation time: 5 minutes

Cooking time: 15 minutes

Servings: 6

Ingredients:

- 1 pound carrots, peeled and thinly sliced
- 2 tablespoons olive oil
- 2 tablespoons curry powder
- 2 tablespoons pure maple syrup juice of ½ lemon
- sea salt
- freshly ground black pepper

Directions:

1. Place the carrots in a large pot and cover with water. Cook on medium-high heat until tender, about 10 minutes. Drain the carrots and return them to the pan over medium-low heat.

2. Stir in the olive oil, curry powder, maple syrup, and lemon juice. Cook, stirring constantly, until the liquid reduces, about 5 minutes. Season with salt and pepper and serve immediately.

Mushroom & Wild Rice Stew

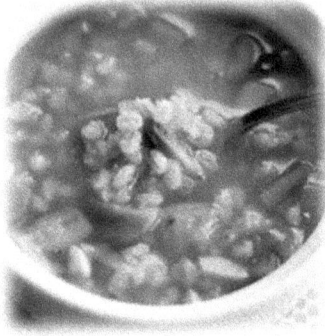

Preparation time: 10 minutes

Cooking time: 50 minutes

Servings: 6

Nutrition: (2 cups)

- Calories: 201
- Protein: 6g
- Total fat: 3g
- Saturated fat: 0g

- Carbohydrates: 44g
- Fiber: 4g

Ingredients:

- 1 to 2 teaspoons olive oil
- 2 cups chopped mushrooms
- ½ to 1 teaspoon salt
- 1 onion, chopped, or 1 teaspoon onion powder
- 3 or 4 garlic cloves, minced, or ½ teaspoon garlic powder
- 1 tablespoon dried herbs
- ¾ cup brown rice
- ¼ cup wild rice or additional brown rice
- 3 cups water
- 3 cups Economical Vegetable Broth or store-bought broth
- 2 to 4 tablespoons balsamic vinegar (optional)
- Freshly ground black pepper
- 1 cup frozen peas, thawed
- 1 cup unsweetened nondairy milk (optional)
- 1 to 2 cups chopped greens, such as spinach, kale, or chard

Directions:

1. Heat the olive oil in a large soup pot over medium-high heat.

2. Add the mushrooms and a pinch of salt, and sauté for about 4 minutes, until the mushrooms are softened. Add the onion and garlic (if using fresh), and sauté for 1 to 2 minutes more. Stir in the dried herbs (plus the onion powder and/or garlic powder, if using), white or brown rice, wild rice, water, vegetable broth, vinegar (if using), and salt and pepper to taste. Bring to a boil, turn the heat to low, and cover the pot. Simmer the soup for 15 minutes (for white riceor 45 minutes (for brown rice). Turn off the heat and stir in the peas, milk (if using), and greens. Let the greens wilt before serving.

3. Leftovers will keep in an airtight container for up to 1 week in the refrigerator or up to 1 month in the freezer.

Almond Soup with Cardamom

Preparation time: 5 minutes

Cooking time: 35 minutes total: 40minutes

Servings: 4

Ingredients:

- 1 tablespoon olive oil
- 1 medium onion, chopped
- 1 medium russet potato, chopped
- 1 medium red bell pepper, chopped
- 4 cups vegetable broth (homemade, store-bought, or water)
- 1/2 teaspoon ground cardamom
- Salt and freshly ground black pepper
- 1/2 cup almond butter
- 1/4 cup sliced toasted almonds, for garnish

Directions:

1. In a large soup pot, heat the oil over medium heat. Add the onion, potato, and bell pepper. Cover and cook until softened, about 5 minutes. Add the broth, cardamom, and salt and pepper to taste. Bring to a boil, then reduce heat to low and simmer, uncovered, until the vegetables are tender, about 30 minutes.

2. Add the almond butter and puree in the pot with an immersion blender or in a blender or food processor, in batches if necessary, and return to the pot. Reheat over medium heat until hot. Taste, adjusting seasonings if necessary, and add more broth or some soy milk if needed for desired consistency.

3. Ladle the soup into bowls, sprinkle with toasted sliced almonds, and serve.

Easy Corn Chowder

Preparation time: 15 minutes

Cooking time: 15 minutes

Servings: 4

Ingredients:

- 2 tablespoons olive oil or other vegetable oil, such as coconut oil
- 1 onion, chopped
- 1 cup chopped fennel bulb or celery
- 2 carrots, peeled and chopped
- 1 red bell pepper, finely chopped
- ¼ cup all-purpose flour
- 6 cups vegetable stock
- 2 cups fresh or canned corn
- 2 cups cubed red potato
- 1 cup unsweetened almond milk or other unsweetened nut or grain milk

- ½ teaspoon sriracha sauce or chili paste (optional sea salt)
- freshly ground black pepper

Directions:

1. In a large pot, heat the olive oil over medium-high heat until it shimmers.
2. Add the onion, fennel, carrots, and bell pepper and cook, stirring occasionally, until the vegetables soften, about 3 minutes.
3. Sprinkle the flour over the vegetables and continue to cook, stirring constantly, for about 2 minutes.
4. Stir in the vegetable stock, using a spoon to scrape any bits of flour or vegetables from the bottom of the pan. Continue stirring until the liquid comes to a boil and the soup begins to thicken. Lower the heat to medium.
5. Add the corn, potatoes, almond milk, and Sriracha, if using. Simmer until the potatoes are soft, about 10 minutes. Season with salt and pepper. Serve hot.

Tamarind Chickpea Stew

Preparation time: 5 minutes

Cooking time: 60 minutes

Servings: 4

Ingredients:

- 1 tablespoon olive oil 1 large onion, chopped
- 2 medium Yukon Gold potatoes, peeled and cut into 1/4-inch dice
- 3 cups cooked chickpeas or 2 (15.5-ouncecans chickpeas, drained and rinsed
- 1 28-ounce can crushed tomatoes
- 1 4-ouncecan mild chopped green chiles, drained
- 2 tablespoons tamarind paste
- 1/4 cup pure maple syrup
- 1 cup vegetable broth, homemade or water
- 2 tablespoons chili powder
- 1 teaspoon ground coriander
- 1/2 teaspoon ground cumin

- Salt and freshly ground black pepper
- 1 cup frozen baby peas, thawed

Directions:

1. In a large saucepan, heat the oil over medium heat. Add the onion, cover, and cook until softened, about 5 minutes. Add the potatoes, chickpeas, tomatoes, and chiles and simmer, uncovered, for 5 minutes.

2. In a small bowl, combine the tamarind paste, maple syrup, and broth and blend until smooth. Stir the tamarind mixture into the vegetables, along with the chili powder, coriander, cumin, and salt and pepper to taste. Bring to a boil, then reduce the heat to medium and simmer, covered, until the potatoes are tender, about 40 minutes.

3. Taste, adjusting seasonings if necessary, and stir in the peas. Simmer, uncovered, about 10 minutes longer. Serve immediately.

Creamy Garlic Mushrooms with Angel Hair Shirataki

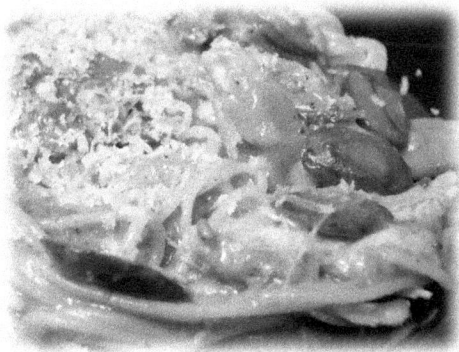

Preparation time: 25 minutes

Serving: 4

Nutritional Values (Per Serving):

- Calories:89
- Total Fat:6.4 g
- Saturated Fat:1.5 g
- Total Carbs: 2g

- Dietary Fiber:0g
- Sugar:1g
- Protein:6 g
- Sodium: 406mg

Ingredients:

For the mushroom sauce:

- 1 tbsp olive oil
- 1 lb chopped mushrooms
- Salt and black pepper to taste 2 tbsp unsalted butter
- garlic cloves, minced
- ½ cup dry white wine
- 1 ½ cups coconut cream
- ½ cup grated parmesan cheese
- 2 tbsp chopped fresh parsley

For the angel hair shirataki:

- 2 (8 oz) packs angel hair shirataki noodles
- Salt to season

Directions:

For the mushroom sauce:

1. Heat the olive oil in a large skillet, season the mushroom with salt and black pepper, and cook in the oil until softened, 5 minutes. Transfer to a plate and set aside.
2. Melt the butter in the skillet and sauté the garlic until fragrant. Stir in the white wine and cook until reduced by half, meanwhile, scraping the bottom of the pan to deglaze.
3. Reduce the heat to low and stir in the coconut cream. Allow simmering for 1 minute and stir in the parmesan cheese to melt.
4. Return the mushroom to the sauce and sprinkle the parsley on top. Adjust the taste with salt and black pepper, if needed.

For the angel hair shirataki:

1. Bring 2 cups of water to a boil in a medium pot over medium heat.
2. Strain the shirataki pasta through a colander and rinse very well under hot running water.
3. Allow proper draining and pour the shirataki pasta into the boiling water. Cook for 3 minutes and strain again.

4. Place a dry skillet over medium heat and stir-fry the shirataki pasta until visibly dry and makes a squeaky sound when stirred, 1 to 2 minutes.
5. Season with salt and plate.
6. Top the shirataki pasta with the mushroom sauce and serve warm.

Golden Couscous Salad

Preparation time: 5 minutes

Cooking time: 12 minutes

Servings: 4

Ingredients:

- 1/4 cup olive oil
- 1 medium shallot, minced
- 1/2 teaspoon ground coriander
- 1/2 teaspoon turmeric
- 1/4 teaspoon ground cayenne
- 1 cup couscous
- 2 cups vegetable broth, homemade or store-bought, or water
- Salt
- 1 medium yellow bell pepper, chopped
- 1 medium carrot, shredded

- ½ cup chopped dried apricots
- ¼ cup golden raisins
- ¼ cup chopped unsalted roasted cashews
- 1½ cups cooked or 1 (15.5-ouncecan chickpeas, drained and rinsed
- 2 tablespoons minced fresh cilantro leaves
- 2 tablespoons fresh lemon juice

Directions:

1. In a large saucepan, heat 1 tablespoon of the oil over medium heat. Add the shallot, coriander, turmeric, cayenne, and couscous and stir until fragrant, about 2 minutes, being careful not to burn. Stir in the broth and salt to taste. Bring to a boil, then remove from the heat, cover, and let stand for 10 minutes.
2. Transfer the cooked couscous to a large bowl. Add the bell pepper, carrot, apricots, raisins, cashews, chickpeas, and cilantro. Toss gently to combine and set aside.
3. In a small bowl, combine the remaining 3 tablespoons of oil with the lemon juice, stirring to blend. Pour the dressing over the salad, toss gently to combine, and serve.

Chopped Salad

Preparation time: 15 minutes

Cooking time: 0 minutes

Servings: 4

Ingredients:

- ¾ cup olive oil
- ¼ cup white wine vinegar
- 2 teaspoons Dijon mustard
- 1 garlic clove
- 1 tablespoon minced green onions
- ½ teaspoon salt (optional)
- ¼ teaspoon ground black pepper
- ½ small head romaine lettuce, chopped
- ½ small head iceberg lettuce, chopped
- 1½ cups cooked or 1 (15.5-ouncecan chickpeas, drained and rinsed
- 2 ripe tomatoes, cut into ½-inch dice

- 1 medium English cucumber, peeled, halved lengthwise, and chopped
- 2 celery ribs, chopped celery
- 1 medium carrot, chopped
- ½ cup halved pitted kalamata olives
- 3 small red radishes, chopped
- 2 tablespoons chopped fresh parsley
- 1 ripe Hass avocado, pitted, peeled, and cut into ½-inch dice

Directions:

1. In a blender or food processor, combine the oil, vinegar, mustard, garlic, green onions, salt, and pepper. Blend well and set aside.
2. In a large bowl, combine the romaine and iceberg lettuces. Add the chickpeas, tomatoes, cucumber, celery, carrot, olives, radishes, parsley, and avocado. Add enough dressing to lightly coat. Toss gently to combine and serve.

Warm Lentil Salad with Red Wine Vinaigrette

Preparation time: 10 minutes

Cooking time: 50 minutes

Servings: 4

Nutrition:

- Calories: 387
- Total fat: 17g
- Carbs: 42g
- Fiber: 19g
- Protein: 18g

Ingredients:

- 1 teaspoon olive oil plus ¼ cup, divided, or 1 tablespoon vegetable broth or water
- 1 small onion, diced

- 1 garlic clove, minced
- 1 carrot, diced
- 1 cup lentils
- 1 tablespoon dried basil
- 1 tablespoon dried oregano
- tablespoon red wine or balsamic vinegar (optional)
- 2 cups water
- ¼ cup red wine vinegar or balsamic vinegar
- 1 teaspoon sea salt
- cups chopped Swiss chard
- 2 cups torn red leaf lettuce
- tablespoons Cheesy Sprinkle

Directions:

1. Heat 1 teaspoon of the oil in a large pot on medium heat, then sauté the onion and garlic until they are translucent, about 5 minutes.
2. Add the carrot and sauté until it is slightly cooked, about 3 minutes. Stir in the lentils, basil, and oregano, then add the wine or balsamic vinegar (if using).
3. Pour the water into the pot and turn the heat up to high to bring to a boil.

4. Turn the heat down to a simmer and let the lentils cook, uncovered, 20 to 30 minutes, until they are soft but not falling apart.

5. While the lentils are cooking, whisk together the red wine vinegar, olive oil, and salt in a small bowl and set aside. Once the lentils have cooked, drain any excess liquid and stir in most of the red wine vinegar dressing. Set a little bit of dressing aside. Add the Swiss chard to the pot and stir it into the lentils. Leave the heat on low and cook, stirring, for at least 10 minutes. Toss the lettuce with the remaining dressing. Place some lettuce on a plate, and top with the lentil mixture. Finish the plate off with a little Cheesy Sprinkle and enjoy.

Carrot and Orange Salad with Cashews and Cilantro

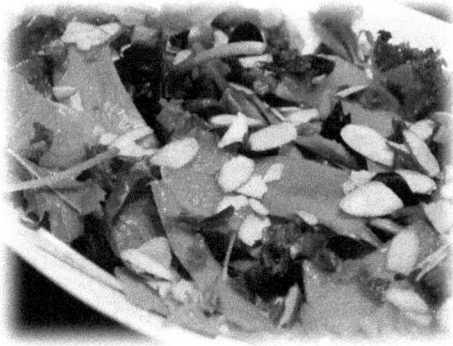

Preparation time: 15 minutes

Cooking time: 0 minutes

Servings: 4

Ingredients:

- 1 pound carrots, shredded
- 2 oranges, peeled, segmented, and chopped
- 1/2 cup unsalted roasted cashews
- 1/4 cup chopped fresh cilantro
- 2 tablespoons fresh orange juice

- 2 tablespoons fresh lime juice
- 2 teaspoons brown sugar (optional9
- Salt (optional) and freshly ground black pepper
- 1/3 cup olive oil

Directions:

1. In a large bowl, combine the carrots, oranges, cashews, and cilantro and set aside.

2. In a small bowl, combine the orange juice, lime juice, sugar, and salt and pepper to taste. Whisk in the oil until blended. Pour the dressing over the carrot mixture, stirring to lightly coat. Taste, adjusting seasonings if necessary. Toss gently to combine and serve.

Kale Chips

Preparation time: 5 minutes

Cooking time: 25 minutes

Servings: 2

Nutritional Values (Per Serving):

- Calories: 144
- Fat: 7g
- Protein: 5g
- Carbohydrates: 18g
- Fiber: 3g
- Sugar: 0g
- Sodium: 363mg

Ingredients:

- 1 large bunch kale

- 1 tablespoon extra-virgin olive oil
- ½ teaspoon chipotle powder
- ½ teaspoon smoked paprika
- ¼ teaspoon salt

Directions:

1. Preheat the oven to 275°F.
2. Line a large baking sheet with parchment paper. In a large bowl, stem the kale and tear it into bite-size pieces. Add the olive oil, chipotle powder, smoked paprika, and salt.
3. Toss the kale with tongs or your hands, coating each piece well.
4. Spread the kale over the parchment paper in a single layer.
5. Bake for 25 minutes, turning halfway through, until crisp.
6. Cool for 10 to 15 minutes before dividing and storing in 2 airtight containers.

Tempeh-Pimiento Cheeze Ball

Preparation time: 5 minutes

Cooking time: 30 minutes

Servings: 8

Ingredients:

- 8 ounces tempeh, cut into 1⁄2-inch pieces
- 1 (2-ouncejar chopped pimientos, drained
- 1⁄4 cup nutritional yeast
- 1⁄4 cup vegan mayonnaise, homemade or store-bought
- 2 tablespoons soy sauce
- 3⁄4 cup chopped pecans

Directions:

1. In a medium saucepan of simmering water, cook the tempeh for 30 minutes. Set aside to cool. In a food processor, combine the cooled tempeh, pimientos,

nutritional yeast, mayo, and soy sauce. Process until smooth.

2. Transfer the tempeh mixture to a bowl and refrigerate until firm and chilled, at least 2 hours or overnight.

3. In a dry skillet, toast the pecans over medium heat until lightly toasted, about 5 minutes. Set aside to cool.

4. Shape the tempeh mixture into a ball, and roll it in the pecans, pressing the nuts slightly into the tempeh mixture so they stick. Refrigerate for at least 1 hour before serving. If not using right away, cover and keep refrigerated until needed. Properly stored, it will keep for 2 to 3 days.

Peppers and Hummus

Preparation time: 15 minutes

Cooking time: 0 minutes

Servings: 4

Ingredients:

- one 15-ounce can chickpeas, drained and rinsed
- juice of 1 lemon, or 1 tablespoon prepared lemon juice
- ¼ cup tahini
- 3 tablespoons olive oil
- ½ teaspoon ground cumin
- 1 tablespoon water
- ¼ teaspoon paprika
- 1 red bell pepper, sliced
- 1 green bell pepper, sliced
- 1 orange bell pepper, sliced

Directions:

1. In a food processor, combine chickpeas, lemon juice, tahini, 2 tablespoons of the olive oil, the cumin, and water.
2. Process on high speed until blended, about 30 seconds. Scoop the hummus into a bowl and drizzle with the remaining tablespoon of olive oil. Sprinkle with paprika and serve with sliced bell peppers.

Deconstructed Hummus Pitas

Preparation time: 15 minutes

Cooking time: 0 minutes

Servings: 4 pitas

Ingredients:

- 1 garlic clove, crushed
- ¾ cup tahini (sesame paste)
- 2 tablespoons fresh lemon juice
- 1 teaspoon salt
- 1/8 teaspoon ground cayenne
- ¼ cup water
- 1½ cups cooked or 1 (15.5-ouncecan chickpeas, rinsed and drained
- 2 medium carrots, grated (about 1 cup)
- 4 (7-inchpita breads, preferably whole wheat, halved
- 1 large ripe tomato, cut into ¼-inch slices
- 2 cups fresh baby spinach

Directions:

1. In a blender or food processor, mince the garlic. Add the tahini, lemon juice, salt, cayenne, and water. Process until smooth.
2. Place the chickpeas in a bowl and crush slightly with a fork. Add the carrots and the reserved tahini sauce and toss to combine. Set aside.
3. Spoon 2 or 3 tablespoons of the chickpea mixture into each pita half. Tuck a tomato slice and a few spinach leaves into each pocket and serve.

Savory Roasted Chickpeas

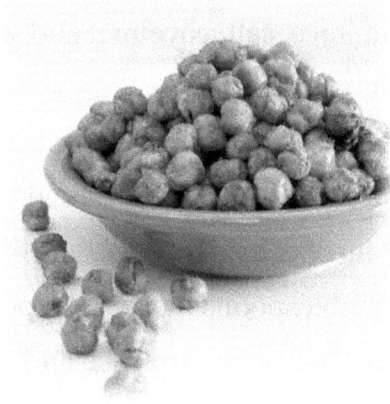

Preparation time: 5 minutes

Cooking time: 25 minutes

Servings: 1 cup

Nutrition (¼ cup)

- Calories: 121
- Total fat: 2g
- Carbs: 20g
- Fiber: 6g
- Protein: 8g

Ingredients:

- 1 (14-ouncecan chickpeas, rinsed and drained, or 1½ cups cooked
- 2 tablespoons tamari, or soy sauce
- 1 tablespoon nutritional yeast
- 1 teaspoon smoked paprika, or regular paprika
- 1 teaspoon onion powder
- ½ teaspoon garlic powder

Directions:

1. Preheat the oven to 400°F.
2. Toss the chickpeas with all the other ingredients, and spread them out on a baking sheet. Bake for 20 to 25 minutes, tossing halfway through.
3. Bake these at a lower temperature, until fully dried and crispy, if you want to keep them longer.
4. You can easily double the batch, and if you dry them out they will keep about a week in an airtight container.

Pumpkin Pie Cups (Pressure cooker)

Preparation time: 5 minutes

Servings: 4-6

Nutrition:

- Calories: 129
- Total fat: 1g
- Protein: 3g
- Sodium: 39mg
- Fiber: 3g

Ingredients:

- 1 cup canned pumpkin purée
- 1 cup nondairy milk

- 6 tablespoons unrefined sugar or pure maple syrup (less if using sweetened milk), plus more for sprinkling
- ¼ cup spelt flour or all-purpose flour
- ½ teaspoon pumpkin pie spice
- Pinch salt

Directions:

1. In a medium bowl, stir together the pumpkin, milk, sugar, flour, pumpkin pie spice, and salt. Pour the mixture into 4 heat-proof ramekins. Sprinkle a bit more sugar on the top of each, if you like. Put a trivet in the bottom of your electric pressure cooker's cooking pot and pour in a cup or two of water. Place the ramekins onto the trivet, stacking them if needed (3 on the bottom, 1 on top).

2. High pressure for 6 minutes. Close and lock the lid and ensure the pressure valve is sealed, then select High Pressure and set the time for 6 minutes.

3. Pressure Release. Once the cook time is complete, quick release the pressure, being careful not to get your fingers or face near the steam release. Once all the pressure has released, carefully unlock and remove the lid. Let cool for a few minutes before carefully lifting out the ramekins

with oven mitts or tongs. Let cool for at least 10 minutes before serving.

Coconut and Almond Truffles

Preparation time: 15 minutes

Cooking time: 0 minutes

Servings: 8 truffles

Ingredients:

- 1 cup pitted dates
- 1 cup almonds
- ½ cup sweetened cocoa powder, plus extra for coating
- ½ cup unsweetened shredded coconut
- ¼ cup pure maple syrup
- 1 teaspoon vanilla extract
- 1 teaspoon almond extract
- ¼ teaspoon sea salt

Directions:

1. In the bowl of a food processor, combine all the ingredients and process until smooth. Chill the mixture for about 1 hour.
2. Roll the mixture into balls and then roll the balls in cocoa powder to coat.
3. Serve immediately or keep chilled until ready to serve.

Pecan and Date-Stuffed Roasted Pears

Preparation time: 10 minutes

Cooking time: 30 minutes

Servings: 4

Ingredients:

- 4 firm ripe pears, cored
- 1 tablespoon fresh lemon juice
- 1⁄2 cup finely chopped pecans
- 4 dates, pitted and chopped
- 1 tablespoon vegan margarine
- 1 tablespoon pure maple syrup
- 1⁄4 teaspoon ground cinnamon
- 1⁄8 teaspoon ground ginger
- 1⁄2 cup pear, white grape, or apple juice

Directions:

1. Preheat the oven to 350°F. Grease a shallow baking dish and set aside. Halve the pears lengthwise and use a melon baller to scoop out the cores. Rub the exposed part of the pears with the lemon juice to avoid discoloration.
2. In a medium bowl, combine the pecans, dates, margarine, maple syrup, cinnamon, and ginger and mix well.
3. Stuff the mixture into the centers of the pear halves and arrange them in the prepared baking pan. Pour the juice over the pears. Bake until tender, 30 to 40 minutes. Serve warm.

Almond Balls

Preparation time: 10 minutes

Cooking time: 0 minutes

Servings: 6

Nutritional Values (Per Serving):

- Calories 194
- Fat 21.2
- Fiber 0.7
- Carbs 1
- Protein 1.4

Ingredients:

- ½ cup coconut oil, melted
- 5 tablespoons almonds, chopped
- 1 tablespoon stevia
- ¼ cup coconut flesh, unsweetened and shredded

Directions:

1. In a bowl, combine the coconut oil with the almonds and the other ingredients, stir well and spoon into round moulds.
2. Serve them cold.

Grapefruit Cream

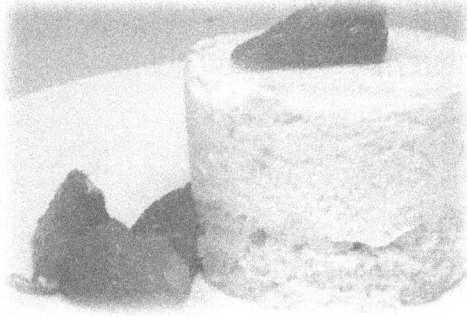

Preparation time: 10 minutes

Cooking time: 0 minutes

Servings: 4

Nutritional Values (Per Serving):

- Calories 346
- Fat 35.5
- Fiber 0
- Carbs 3.4
- Protein 4.6

Ingredients:

- 2 cups coconut cream
- 1 cup grapefruit, peeled, and chopped
- 2 tablespoons stevia
- 1 teaspoon vanilla extract

Directions:

1. In a blender, combine the coconut cream with the grapefruit and the other ingredients, pulse well, divide into bowls and serve cold.

Tangerine Stew

Preparation time: 10 minutes

Cooking time: 10 minutes

Servings: 4

Nutritional Values (Per Serving):

- calories 289
- fat 26.1
- fiber 3.9
- carbs 10.3
- protein 5.7

Ingredients:

- 1 cup coconut water
- 2 cups tangerines, peeled and cut into segments
- 1 tablespoon lime juice
- 1 tablespoon stevia
- ½ teaspoon vanilla extract

Directions:

2. In a pan, combine the coconut water with the tangerines and the other ingredients, toss, bring to a simmer and cook over medium heat for 10 minutes.
3. Divide into bowls and serve cold.

Creamy Pineapple Mix

Preparation time: 10 minutes

Cooking time: 10 minutes

Servings: 4

Nutritional Values (Per Serving):

- Calories 329
- Fat 32.7
- Fiber 0
- Carbs 2.5
- Protein 5.7

Ingredients:

- 1 teaspoon nutmeg, ground
- 1 cup pineapple, peeled and cubed
- 1 cup coconut cream
- ½ cup stevia
- 1 teaspoon vanilla extract

Directions:

1. In a pan, combine the pineapple with the nutmeg and the other ingredients, toss, cook over medium heat for 10 minutes, divide into bowls and serve.

Avocado and Pineapple Bowls

Preparation time: 10 minutes

Cooking time: 0 minutes

Servings: 4

Nutritional Values (Per Serving):

- Calories 312
- Fat 29.5
- Fiber 3.3
- Carbs 16.7
- Protein 5

Ingredients:

- 2 tablespoons avocado oil
- 1 cup pineapple, peeled and cubed
- 2 avocados, peeled, pitted and cubed
- 2 tablespoons stevia
- Juice of 1 lime

Directions:

1. In a bowl, combine the pineapple with the avocados and the other ingredients, toss, and serve cold.

Pineapple and Melon Stew

Preparation time: 10 minutes

Cooking time: 15 minutes

Servings: 4

Nutritional Values (Per Serving):

- Calories 40
- Fat 4.3
- Fiber 2.3
- Carbs 3.4
- Protein 0.8

Ingredients:

- 2 tablespoons stevia
- 1 cup pineapple, peeled and cubed
- 1 cup melon, peeled and cubed
- 2 cups water
- 1 teaspoon vanilla extract

Directions:

1. In a pan, combine the pineapple with the melon and the other ingredients, toss gently, cook over medium-low heat for 15 minutes, divide into bowls and serve cold.

Roasted Almonds

Preparation time: 5 minutes

Cooking time: 5 minutes

Servings: 4

Nutritions (Per Servings):

- Calories: 342
- Fat: 31.1g
- Sugar: 2.1 g
- Carbohydrates: 11.5 g
- Cholesterol: 0 mg
- Protein: 10.2 g

Ingredients:

- 2 cups almonds, blanched
- 2 tablespoons rosemary

- 1 teaspoon salt
- 2 tablespoons olive oil
- 1 teaspoon paprika

Directions:

1. In a pan over medium-high heat add almonds and heat until toasted. Reduce heat to medium-low and add salt, paprika, and rosemary. Cook almonds for another 3 minutes. Serve immediately and enjoy!

Cheese Fries

Preparation time: 5 minutes

Cooking time: 4 minutes

Servings: 4

Nutritions:

- Calories: 200
- Sugar: 0.3 g
- Fat: 18 g
- Carbohydrates: 1 g
- Cholesterol: 42 mg
- Protein: 12 g

Ingredients:

- 8-ounces halloumi cheese, sliced into fries
- 2-ounces tallow
- 1 serving marinara sauce, low carb

Directions:

1. Heat the tallow in a pan over medium heat. Gently place halloumi pieces in the pan. Cook halloumi fries for 2 minutes on each side or until lightly golden brown. Serve with marinara sauce and enjoy!

Crunchy Parmesan Crisps

Preparation time: 5 minutes

Cooking time: 3 minutes

Servings: 12

Nutritions:

- Calories: 64
- Carbohydrates: 0.7 g
- Sugar: 0 g
- Fat: 4.3 g
- Cholesterol: 14 mg
- Protein: 6.4 g

Ingredients:

- 12 tablespoons Parmesan cheese, shredded

Directions:

1. Preheat your oven to 400° Fahrenheit. Spray a baking tray with cooking spray. Place each tablespoon of cheese on a baking tray. Bake in preheated oven for 3 minutes or until lightly brown. Allow cooling time, serve and enjoy!

Cinnamon Coconut Chips

Preparation time: 5 minutes

Cooking time: 2 minutes

Servings: 2

Nutrtions:

- Calories: 228
- Carbohydrates: 7.8 g
- Fat: 21 g
- Sugar: 0 g
- Cholesterol: 0 mg
- Protein: 1.9 g

Ingredients:

- ¼ cup coconut chips, unsweetened
- ¼ teaspoon sea salt
- ¼ cup cinnamon

Directions:

1. Add cinnamon and salt in a mixing bowl and set aside. Heat a pan over medium heat for 2 minutes. Place the coconut chips in the hot pan and stir until coconut chips crisp and lightly brown. Toss toasted coconut chips with cinnamon and salt. Serve and enjoy!

Roasted Cashews

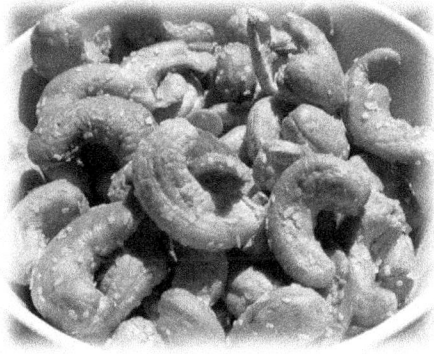

Preparation time: 5 minutes

Cooking time: 3 hours

Servings: 4

Nutritions:

- Calories: 205
- Sugar: 1.8 g
- Fat: 15.9 g
- Carbohydrates: 13.9 g
- Cholesterol: 0 mg
- Protein: 5.4 g

Ingredients:

- 1 cup cashews
- 1 cup water
- 2 tablespoons cinnamon

Directions:

1. Add water and cashews to a bowl and soak overnight. Drain the cashews and place on a paper towel to dry. Preheat oven to 200° Fahrenheit. Place the soaked cashews on a baking tray. Sprinkle cashews with cinnamon. Roast in preheated oven for 3 hours. Allow cooling time and then serve and enjoy!

www.ingramcontent.com/pod-product-compliance
Lightning Source LLC
Chambersburg PA
CBHW050749030426
42336CB00012B/1734